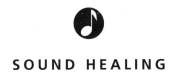

SOUND HEALING

Ease Chronic Pain

Text copyright © 2005 Howard Richman, Judy Nelson

Published in 2005 by
Stewart, Tabori & Chang
115 West 18th Street
New York, NY 10011
www.abramsbooks.com

Library of Congress Cataloging-in-Publication Data
Richman, Howard.
    Sound healing : ease chronic pain / by Howard Richman & Judy Nelson.
        p. cm.
    Includes index.
    ISBN 1-58479-466-6
    1. Music therapy.   I. Nelson, Judy Ellen. II. Title.

ML3920.R53 2005
615.8'5154--dc22

                                                        2005013856

Editor: Debora Yost
Production Manager: Kim Tyner
Designed by Larissa Nowicki

The text of this book was composed in Adobe Frutiger

Printed in China

10 9 8 7 6 5 4 3 2 1

First Printing

Stewart, Tabori & Chang is a subsidiary of LA MARTINIÈRE
GROUPE

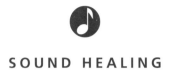

SOUND HEALING

Ease Chronic Pain

MUSIC • IMAGERY • BOOK • JOURNAL

Howard Richman
Composer

Judy Nelson
Music Therapist

STEWART, TABORI & CHANG • NEW YORK

CONTENTS

EASE CHRONIC PAIN CD

Track 1   Listening Instructions · · · · (2:36)

Track 2   Music to Ease Chronic Pain (Piano Solo) · · (24:28)

Track 3   Guided Imagery for Pain Release · · · (29:57)

How to Get the Most from This Program

Not New Age. New Age and meditation music are usually very soothing and calming—what we would call ambient. This means that they are more like calm background music. Music to Ease Chronic Pain is the opposite. It aggressively confronts your pain and then gradually helps to transmute it through the process of transformational entrainment. That's why you should consider it foreground music.

Sound Healing: Ease Chronic Pain offers an alternative and complementary approach to dealing with persistent pain. This book and CD will introduce you to healing music and guided imagery, explain how they work, and help you explore how to use them to promote your own health and well-being.

Sound is all around us, yet we often are unaware of its power to heal. The music and guided imagery on the accompanying CD are works that we've created to help you release your pain and achieve a state of mind/body balance. It is our heartfelt desire to bring sound vibration into your life with its possibilities for healing and transformation.

THERE ARE FOUR PARTS TO THIS PROGRAM:

- A **guidebook** that explains how *Sound Healing: Ease Chronic Pain* works and how to use it most effectively.

- An original piano composition of **healing music** targeted to relieve pain.

- Follow-along **guided imagery**, also originally created for this volume, which will help you experience or "image" your pain and help set it free.

- A **journal** to record your personal experience.

The guidebook is an important part of the program, and we recommend that you read it before listening to the CD in order to get the full benefit of the *Sound Healing* experience. After reading the book and learning how the two healing arts work, you will be ready to listen to the CD. It is important to understand that you do not have to follow the sequence as it is on the CD. You may want to experience the guided imagery before the music, or just do one or the other. After reading this book, however, you will understand why you will achieve the best results from doing both.

We do encourage you to experiment. For example, if you listen to the guided imagery first, it may help to get you into a more receptive state for listening to the healing music.

Or if you first listen to the healing music, and you feel an emotional or physical shift occur, you may find it very powerful to then listen to the guided imagery to help lock in or integrate the experience.

If you are able to follow the listening suggestions, you should have a positive experience on your very first listening! However, just like peeling the layers from an artichoke, each time you listen, you will get closer to your desired outcome. The benefit from each listening should reach deeper and different levels of your pain and become more and more helpful. This is why we recommend that you listen to both the healing music and the guided imagery components every day, once a day, for 30 days. Don't worry if you miss a day, however. You will not lose any of the benefit you have already attained.

After this period, you will be better able to gauge which components are helping you the most. For some, it will be the nonverbal experience of listening to the music. For others, it will be the verbal excursion of the guided imagery. Some people are more verbal/visual and do very well with the guided imagery. Others are more tactile/emotional and do very well with the music listening. It is up to you to personalize this program so you can get the most from it. Explore what combination works best for you.

LISTENING SUGGESTIONS: THE MUSIC

The CD begins with a short introduction. The music begins on track 2. Unlike with typical background music, you need to listen to this healing music responsively—meaning all the way through without interruption. This allows your body to follow through the musical progression that will help lead you to freedom from pain.

Be prepared: You will not be hearing traditional melodies. You may feel this music has no melody at all. Many people do not like the initial "taste" of the music, but they like how they feel after they have heard it! This is because the music was created to be a sound version of pain—a type of sound "mirror" that at first reflects the current stress or turmoil your pain is causing, and by the end, reflects a feeling of pain relief. As the music gradually transforms and as you listen to it again and again, you should be able to experience its resolution both physically and emotionally.

You may reach a point where you think you just can't stand to hear it one more time. You may feel that the initial momentum you built is suddenly being met with a certain resistance. This is not unusual. In fact, it can be good. If this occurs, hang in there anyway. This resistance can be the breakthrough or threshold towards change. So, please, do not give up!

PREPARING YOUR ENVIRONMENT

Ideally, you should listen to the music through speakers rather than headphones so that the very cells of your body can listen to and feel the sound. (If you only have headphones, this will still be okay.) Arrange your listening environment so that you are as comfortable as possible. Take off your shoes. Stand at ease, sit, or lie down. Take a few deep breaths to help you relax.

Allow the music to penetrate your body and reach your inner feeling. Respond to it freely. Everyone has a different manner of expression. You may experience visual images, thoughts, movement, an intensification of emotion, physical vibrations, sleep, or nothing at all. Remember, your honest response to the music is what is important. Your reaction to the music is what helps trigger a release of the emotional/cellular memory, where you store the memory of your pain.

Listen actively rather than passively. Do not think that you have to just stay still and concentrate on the music. In fact, if the music inspires you to get up and do something or if your mind begins to wander, allow, allow, allow! Accept all responses without concern. On the other hand, do not begin listening to the music while you are already doing other unrelated activities. Remember, this is not intended as background music. You must let the music embrace you totally.

When the music stops, bask in the silence for many moments. This will help integrate the feelings that surfaced during the previous 25 minutes. It can take several listenings before you feel you are making progress. This is where the book's journal comes in. Writing down your feelings after each session will help you remember your path to wellness and hopefully will allow you to better understand your pain.

LISTENING SUGGESTIONS: GUIDED IMAGERY

The third track takes you from healing music to guided imagery, a technique in which you use the mind's eye to help move the pain out of your body. It is intended to evoke a feeling of calm and to relax the nervous system to facilitate pain relief. The complete text of the imagery can be found on page 84, if you wish to read it first. But it is not necessary.

You will be introduced to visualizations that will help you see your pain as an energy that you can overcome and banish from your body. We encourage you to listen to the guided imagery many times and as often as desired, especially if this is a technique that is new to you. Each time you listen enhances your visualization experience and deepens the calming response in your nervous system.

Do not be concerned if you do not feel a change in your pain after doing the visualization for the first time, or even the first few times. You may not be able to fully relax or prevent your thoughts from wandering. This is okay. Be patient and proceed at whatever pace works for you.

PREPARING YOUR ENVIRONMENT

Your listening environment should be free from distraction and interruptions, such as telephones, television, and family. It should have a comfortable chair. Loosen your belt or any clothing that is restrictive. This will help make it easier for you to reach a state of relaxation.

Sit down, take off your shoes, and place your feet flat on the floor. Your feet are integral to the process because they keep you centered in your body. Try to keep them flat on the floor throughout the entire imagery exercise. Place your palms face up on top of your thighs. This is important as well because you will feel a release of pain energy leaving your body through the palms of your hands.

Whether you are listening through stereo headphones or speakers make sure to keep it at a comfortable, "conversational" volume.

Keep your attention focused on the voice and what it is telling you to do. You might have a hard time with focus at first, but follow the imagery through from start to finish. If your mind strays, gently bring yourself back to the guided imagery. If you are unable to, just let it go off on its own. Follow your inner voice and see where it leads you.

The guided imagery is an opportunity for you to create space and time in your life just for you. It is your time to take care of yourself. Recognize how supportive and validating it is to give yourself this time for pain release, rejuvenation, and relaxation.

LET YOUR FEELINGS SURFACE

While following along, you may begin to feel emotions surface from your unconscious mind. This is natural and always a good sign. It may be a signal that an energy is being released that contributed to your emotional, psychological, and physical stress.

Do not suppress any feelings that might surface into your conscious mind. Observe each feeling as an envelope—inside the envelope is a message from your unconscious mind to your conscious mind. The message is about healing your pain. Sometimes these messages are about letting go of pent-up feelings and old beliefs that do not serve to create a balanced and healthy state of being. Sometimes they are about making changes in your life. Do not feel as though you need to make these changes immediately, as that could add to your stress. Let the imagery guide you through releasing all these feelings.

THE JOURNAL

Use the journal starting on page 64 to learn more about your experience with healing music and guided imagery. We suggest that you take 5 minutes after listening to the CD to think about your experience and record your thoughts. Allow yourself to freely express what you are feeling physically, mentally, emotionally, and spiritually. Write about your realizations, and explore what they mean in relationship to you and your life.

To help get you get started, we offer a few exercises to spark your creativity. They are only suggestions. It is quite all right to create your journal in any form you desire.

Pain often comes in cycles. When chronic pain goes away, we tend to become tense with anxiety that it will return. This can actually create more pain! When the body tenses, it releases stress hormones that signal the brain to begin another pain cycle.

By learning to relax, it is possible to break the pain cycle. This is one of the valuable benefits of guided imagery. There are many things in life that make us tense. For someone with pain, constant tension can make it intensify, and make it harder to get rid of or control. One of the goals in your pain-management program should be to identify your personal stressors. It can be tricky to get rid of them because you don't always recognize that they exist. Here are some suggestions to help get rid of stress:

Learn to say "no." Force yourself to stop taking on more projects than you can comfortably do. It often seems that you are "the only one" who can make something happen. If you have the fortitude to say "no," someone else will come along who can do the task.

Take time for yourself. Even if you are a natural "giver," you won't have much to give if your resources are depleted. Every day, spend a little time doing something nurturing for yourself. This could be taking a walk, reading, taking a bath, meditating, listening to music (and guided imagery), laughing, or just enjoying the moment.

The obvious things, such as taking a vacation or getting a massage, can be relaxing but require scheduling, which can add to the tension. It's better to find little things that encourage relaxation throughout the day so that it becomes part of your lifestyle.

Be aware of the state of your body during normal activities. When you're eating, do you raise your shoulders more than necessary? When you're driving, is your left foot tense for no reason? When you're watching TV, are you squinting? These little "wasted energy" events add up to overall tension, and this can lead to pain.

Music as Healer

Judy Nelson

• • • • • • • • • • •

SOUND HEALING HISTORY

In primitive cultures, illness was viewed as being caused by angry spirits or evil magic. Musical instruments were thought to have magical properties. How else could a hollow piece of wood poked with holes produce such an achingly beautiful sound?

Our ancestors may have viewed these sounds as voices or spirits within the instruments themselves. It took a specialist, called a shaman, to play the instruments that would conjure up the spirits for appeasing and healing the sick and wounded.

In ancient Africa, special songs, instruments, and dances were combined with healing rituals to treat the sick. Instruments, such as the drum and the harp, were believed to have healing powers and were played over the afflicted area to bring about a cure.

Ancient Greeks had a keen interest in the power of music to heal. They studied the effects of scales and rhythms on mood and health, and began to systematically apply music as a treatment for the sick.

As a music therapist, I have had many opportunities to witness the healing power of music. While I was the director of music therapy at a Los Angeles hospital that treats seriously ill people, I was awed by the power of music to override the need for morphine during severe states of pain. I was touched when the last thing a dying soul heard was his favorite music. I felt privileged to be the messenger of such a healing art.

One patient was a man, whom I will call Tony, in his mid-forties with the blood defect known as hemophilia. Tony also had the AIDS virus from a transfusion he received before blood was routinely screened. Tony was in and out of the hospital over the course of a year for treatment due to a variety of infections and health complications. As his health started to deteriorate, his pain began to increase.

Tony loved music, so I supplied him with a variety of musical recordings that he could listen to when his pain was at its highest level, which was during the evening and during physical therapy. I brought in my guitar and hand drums, and we created live music in his hospital room. Tony's smile lit up the whole room when there was music present. He told me that music had brought him quality of life and a lot of joy during his difficult journey with an incurable disease.

On the pediatric unit of the same hospital, I worked at different times with two teenage girls with sickle-cell anemia, another rare, incurable, and painful hereditary disease. The girls experienced acutely painful episodes during which they were hospitalized and attached to morphine drips. Their pain was so intense that at times they were in the hospital for as long as two weeks, which gave me ample opportunity to create music experiences with them. I used a music synthesizer to engage the girls in writing songs, playing keyboard, and singing. I designed for each of them a music-listening program consisting of their favorite music inserted between music I selected to reduce their stress and help them relax. With both girls, I noticed that when I engaged them in music, they pushed the button on their morphine drip about every hour. When I visited them without the benefit of music, they pushed their morphine buttons about every 15 minutes. The experience of making or listening to music directed their attention away from their pain, thereby reducing the need to self-administer morphine.

Another patient I worked with was a woman in her sixties undergoing chemotherapy for cancer. I'll call her Sonia. I was consulted because Sonia was experiencing a great deal of discomfort due to nausea, and her doctor thought music might help to minimize pain. Sonia and I designed a music-listening program based on the rate, intensity, and timing of the physical symptoms she experienced during chemotherapy. During the first stage of treatment, Sonia felt symptoms of anxiety, such as an elevated heart rate and shallow breathing. She had a fear of the nausea and pain she often experienced during chemotherapy. I used a principle of music therapy called the "iso" principle, in which the music is designed to "match" the pain and "move" it to a state of less, and then no, pain.

I started Sonia with a short excerpt of energetic music from her favorite movie soundtrack, then a short excerpt of a medium-tempo pop song, followed by a long, slow movement from her favorite classical composition.

During the next stage of treatment, Sonia felt lethargic, so the music chosen reflected slow tempos that felt soothing to her. The most difficult stage of treatment was when Sonia felt nauseated, so two hours of her rock/pop favorites were stacked by the CD player on her nightstand so she could listen to them one after another. After the nausea subsided, Sonia preferred to listen to either classical music or the rest of her favorite movie soundtrack.

Sonia told her doctors that with the aid of the healing music, she experienced less anxiety, pain, and nausea during treatment. The music-listening program was a success.

Tony, Sonia, and the teenage girls all experienced less pain and discomfort as a result of listening to music. They also reported that making music and listening to music gave them emotional support.

THE PROOF IS IN

These are just three stories out of hundreds that I have personally witnessed. Thousands of music therapists from around the world have had these experiences, too. The names and faces change, but the story remains the same: Music heals. And the evidence isn't just anecdotal. Hundreds of studies have been conducted around the world that validate music as a healing therapy. For example:

- At the University of Miami pain clinic, patients were exposed to one-hour music-listening sessions once a week for ten weeks. They listened to music while resting comfortably in a recliner. Music was chosen according to their ages and individual preferences. While the patients listened to the music, researchers monitored changes in heart rate, skin temperature, and muscle activity. After the study, the patients reported that the music helped them relax more deeply, not only when they listened to it, but also when they felt tense during the day and mentally recalled the music. Approximately 70 percent of the patients were able to decrease their pain medication. The patients also reported that music helped make them feel optimistic and improved their outlook on life.

- In another study at a regional university in southern Alabama, undergraduate psychology students were measured for the effects of music on anxiety. Students were asked to complete two questionnaires, then either listen to music or sit in silence for about a half hour, complete two more questionnaires, and then take a difficult and stressful mental-task test. During the test, the students sat in a recliner attached to biofeedback sensors that measured heart rate, skin temperature, and muscle activity.

  The students were divided into three music-listening groups: classical, rock music, and music of their preference. A fourth group did not listen to any music. In addition to the biofeedback measurements, students rated themselves on feelings of anxiety before and after the task. Those who listened to music that they personally selected reported having the greatest feelings of relaxation.They, along with those who listened to classical music, also had less anxiety.

- A study at the Spinal Pain Clinic in Dallas investigated how different types of music and imagery affected patients' perception of pain. Twenty-three people with spinal pain were divided into two groups. One group received guided imagery with music, and the other group received imagery without music. The imagery focused on pain being subdued by the body's natural endorphins, the "feel-good" hormones. Researchers found that those who listened to music combined with imagery experienced deeper relaxation and less pain than the patients who heard guided imagery without music.

- Researchers demonstrated music's powerful effect on the immune system in a study that divided 36 students into two groups: a music group and a nonmusic group. Both groups gave blood samples to measure levels of the hormones interleukin-1 and cortisol. Interleukin-1 is an immune-boosting hormone and cortisol is a stress hormone. Both naturally occur in the body. After giving a blood sample, one group listened to relaxing music for about 15 minutes. The other group did not listen to music. Blood samples were taken again at the end of the 15 minutes. Both groups completed an anxiety questionnaire after the first blood sample and before the final blood sample. Results showed that the group that listened to relaxing music had significantly higher levels of the immune-boosting hormone and significantly lower levels of the stress hormone than the group that did not listen to the music.

- Music can also have a positive influence on the emotional stress of the terminally ill. In one study, 40 nursing home residents participated in music activities such as singing, playing instruments, writing songs, and doing vocal and rhythmic improvisations, and 40 others did not. Results showed that those who participated in music lived longer and were able to engage in music activities even when they felt agitated or no longer able to verbally communicate. Other studies of home hospice centers reported similar results.

- A study at the Chronic Pain Rehabilitation Unit of the Golden Valley Health Center in Minneapolis found that music helped increase the activity level and outlook on life among patients with chronic pain.

Patients participated in 60-minute sessions daily that included 15 minutes of exercises and 45 minutes of group activities including recreation, crafts, and discussions on positive coping strategies all accompanied by music. During the activities, the music therapist reinforced positive statements and ignored negative comments. As a result, most of the participants increased their activity levels. They even requested that music continue to be played during their exercise sessions and also during leisure hours.

Music has also been shown to significantly decrease pain perception in a variety of situations, from the anxiety associated with going to the dentist, to foot pain, to the side effects of chemotherapy, to severe burns. Studies have also shown that music is effective in reducing pain perception during childbirth labor and after surgery.

A WHOLE-BODY EXPERIENCE

You may not realize it, but you have already experienced the healing power of music many times in your own life. You experience it every time you turn on the radio and say to yourself, *I love this song!* Music has the ability to move us on every level. Physically, music can make us get up and dance or sit back and relax. Mentally, music can catch our attention by the unexpected chord or song lyric. Emotionally, music can make us laugh or bring us to tears. Spiritually, it can move us to states of rapture.

Indeed, music is a whole-body experience. It has the ability to get to the very core of our being. No one demonstrated this better than a guy I'll call Joe, who often came to a nightclub where I perform. One night while I was singing, I noticed him on the dance floor moving to the music and having a great time.

When I took my break, I went around the club to greet regulars, as I usually do, and introduced myself to Joe. I found out that Joe is profoundly deaf and communicates through sign language. Though he could not hear, Joe was wearing a large hearing aid behind each ear that received sound vibration and delivered it to the inner ear through his skull bone in order to stimulate his auditory nerve. He explained that he thoroughly enjoyed experiencing and dancing to music even though he could not perceive music in the same way a hearing person does. Joe described the sensation of listening to music as feeling the vibration of the sound in his feet; it then moved throughout his body, allowing him to follow the pulse of the music. Joe indicated that even though he was deaf, the music made his body want to dance. He enjoyed being around live music, and going to clubs to follow his favorite bands was an important part of his life. Joe has become a regular at my club gigs over the years, and it is still a joy to see him out on the dance floor. He reminds me that music is something to be felt as well as heard.

SOUND IS ENERGY

Sound is created by energy acting upon a material, which causes the material to vibrate. In the case of the human voice, it is the vocal cords that vibrate as air is pushed through them while traveling up from the lungs. In some musical instruments, vibration occurs as energy acts upon a string, as with a guitar, or a stretched skin, as with a drum. In other musical instruments, vibration occurs when energy acts upon the air within a tube, such as a flute or a pipe organ.

As vibration occurs, the movement to and fro disturbs molecules within and around the space of the pulsating material, creating energy waves that travel molecule by molecule to the human ear. These waves of energy reach the ear, which is naturally shaped to collect them, funnel them into the ear canal, and deliver them to the eardrum. The eardrum, which separates the ear canal from the middle ear, vibrates like the stretched skin of a drum when it is struck. When the eardrum vibrates, it causes a chain reaction among three tiny bones within the middle ear and hair cells within the inner ear that send signals along the auditory nerve to the brain to be processed and understood. The sensitive hair cells of the inner ear are responsible for encoding all that you hear—the volume, the pitch, and the duration of sound.

While your ear is collecting sound waves and funneling them toward the brain, sound waves are also reaching your whole body. Your skin has receptors that perceive even the most subtle of vibrations—hence, your ability to feel a gentle breeze brush against your cheek. As sound vibrations surround and touch your body, listening to music becomes a whole-body, vibro tactile experience. Music does not need to be extremely loud in order for this to occur. Listening at a comfortable volume is all you need to receive the potential benefits of sound vibration throughout your body.

Music affects the body in a number of ways. Heart rate and breathing tend to get in rhythm with the pulse of the music, so when you listen to music that has a slow tempo, your heartbeat and breathing tend to slow down. Conversely, if you listen to music that has a fast, driving tempo, your heartbeat and breathing will tend to become faster. Since pain can cause physical and emotional stress, you may experience increased muscle tension, faster heartbeat and breathing rates, and higher blood pressure. Listening to music that entrains these systems to operate at a calmer level has been shown to release tension and slow heartbeat and breathing rates. Reduced stress levels help boost the immune system and help return the body to a state of balance.

Music contains many components that individually are not very "musical." Yet together, these elements can form the simplest song to the most complex symphony. It is the combination of these elements that has the power to captivate your body, emotions, and mind.

Pitch. The high-low quality of a musical sound, determined by the frequency of the tone (for example, the number of vibrations per second).

Rhythm. The long and short duration of musical sounds.

Melody. The succession of musical tones forming a line of individual significance and expressive value.

Scale/Mode. A succession of notes arranged in ascending or descending order.

Harmony. The succession and relationship of pitches to one another within a musical composition.

Form. The structure or organization of the music (for example, verse-chorus-verse-chorus).

Tempo. The speed of the beat.

Dynamics. The relative loudness or softness of musical sounds.

Articulation. The connectedness and disconnectedness of notes. There are many articulations but the most common are legato (connected) and staccato (disconnected).

Phrasing. A musical breath.

MUSIC AND THE BRAIN

Your brain is a wonder of nature. It only weighs approximately three pounds, but contains over one hundred billion nerve cells that are capable of receiving and interpreting information in myriad ways. With the use of modern technology such as PET (Positron Emission Tomography) scans, researchers have been able to pinpoint exact locations in the brain that activate a healing response to music. Studies reveal that when you are listening to music, the left hemisphere of the brain processes rhythm, stress and inflection, and the right hemisphere of the brain processes pitch, melody, and volume changes. Within the brain's hemispheres are structures that can be profoundly affected by music.

The spinal cord is like a multi lane highway of nerves leading to and from the brain. Skin, muscles, and internal organs are all connected to the brain by nerves that run through the spinal cord. Signals carrying sensory and movement information are sent along these nerves in milliseconds. Pain travels the same way.

There are two types of responses to sensory information—voluntary and autonomic. Voluntary responses, such as reaching for a pen, are under our control. Many responses are not under our voluntary control and are governed by our autonomic (automatic) nervous system. Autonomic behaviors such as heartbeat, respiration, digestion, and the release of hormones occur without any conscious awareness. The autonomic nervous system is integrally connected to our emotions, and emotions play a large role in our awareness of pain. Research reveals that pain perception increases as feelings of anxiety and stress rise, and conversely, pain perception decreases as such feelings lessen.

HOW MUSIC REPLACES PAIN

All pain transmitted to the brain is first received by a part of the brain called the thalamus. From there it is sent to a place called the somatosensory area where it is processed. The hypothalamus is another key structure of the brain that integrates emotional reactions and the autonomic nervous system.

Below the thalamus and hypothalamus is the midbrain. It contains nuclei and nerve tracts known as the reticular formation. This area assists in controlling body functions such as respiration, circulation, alertness, and sleep cycles. Of particular significance is the fact that listening to music can cause the reticular formation to focus on the music instead of pain sensations.

Researchers generally believe that neurotransmitters in the brain control sensitivity to pain. One such neurotransmitter, serotonin, is released at nerve junctures and can inhibit the strength of the pain signal as it moves along its pathway. Music can activate areas in the brain that release naturally occurring opiates such as endorphins, that have the ability to block pain signals from reaching the brain.

Researchers agree that emotions are tied to our awareness of pain. Emotions such as anxiety, depression, and fear arouse a chemical reaction in various brain structures that can increase the sensation of pain. However, if the brain structures that respond to emotional stress are processing enjoyable music instead, it can result in reduced perception of pain. The less pain you perceive, the more positive you feel.

EMOTIONAL PAIN

Emotional pain can be the most debilitating of all. It dulls our senses, puts us into inner conflict, and can lead us to a feeling of utter anguish. It is in these moments that music can make the biggest difference. Music has the ability to bypass the logical part of our brain and reach directly into our "emotional brain." It can help us connect with hope. Music can envelop our psyche and bathe it in vibrations that shift our thoughts and feelings to new perspectives and possibilities. Music reminds us that we are not alone, that others have felt the way we do, and that there is strength in our common experience. Music is not a substitute for other interventions, but it certainly may become a partner in healing.

How This Music Works

Howard Richman

• • • • • • • • • • •

SOUND HEALING HISTORY

References since biblical times indicate the use of music to heal various afflictions. The Book of I Samuel 16:16-18 makes reference to David playing his lyre to sooth King Saul when he was troubled by an evil spirit. In ancient Egypt, physicians were trained to be musicians in order to use incantations to cure the sick.

In Hawaiian culture, healers known as *kahunas* have an ancient tradition of chanting that focuses on helping the body become enlightened and healthy at the cellular level. Combined with hula dancing, chanting and movement are intended to give the body specific instructions on how to "rearrange" itself to achieve vibrant health.

Native Americans have a rich tradition of using music to heal. Many shamans believed that the power to heal certain diseases or illnesses was contained within a specific song. This belief went so deep that a shaman would not treat a condition unless he felt confident in his knowledge of the proper song. Shamans used singing, chanting, drumming, and dancing without stopping for several days as a way to purge illness.

The music in the *Ease Chronic Pain* CD is different than any music you have ever experienced. Your initial reaction will likely be one of surprise.

We usually think of music as a universal pleasure that helps make life more interesting and fun. It can be energizing, and it can be relaxing. It can be company and comfort when we are alone. It keeps us entertained while we're stalled in traffic, motivates us when we're doing housework, and keeps us moving during exercise. It gets us in the mood for love. Music is in the background of almost every component and emotion of life. Healing music, however, is foreground music.

LIKE MUSIC MEDICINE

When you turn on the radio, you immediately search for the sounds you love. It is like a buddy that lifts your spirit and enhances your mood. But it won't take your physical pain away. Rather, the music that offers the greatest healing benefit is likely music that you would not choose at all. Why? Because it feels too similar to your pain.

Think of it this way: You often take cough medicine because you know it will bring relief from your symptoms and discomfort, even though you don't like the taste. *Music to Ease Chronic Pain* is like music medicine. It is not a taste you recognize or necessarily enjoy, but you try it because you know it will make you feel better.

Don't get me wrong; it *is* music. In fact, people tell me that they look forward to listening to it again and again because they like the way it makes them feel.

GIVE YOURSELF A MUSICAL MASSAGE

Think of *Music to Ease Chronic Pain* as a musical massage. The sound waves themselves have a force that can help relax the blocked energy that may be associated with your pain. Some of the sections of the music are repetitive in nature. This minimalistic approach to repeating a musical pattern may seem odd until you begin to understand and actually feel the hidden benefit. The repetition is intentional in order for the musical passages to resonate in the areas of your being where you have the most pain—just like fingers kneading a sore back during a massage.

As you listen, feel the music going deep into your pain and gently moving it out of your body . . . little by little . . . layer by layer . . . with each musical repetition. Ah-h-h-h-h. Feel the relief!

SOUND MIRROR: A NEW WAY TO SEE PAIN

Gripping, shooting, wandering, piercing, stinging, agonizing. These are just a few of the adjectives people use to describe pain. Not only is pain difficult to endure, it is difficult to describe. And it is just as difficult for someone else to understand. No one can really feel your pain, though saying so is a nice gesture. Music, however, *can* "feel" your pain. Here is how it works:

My healing music is based on a principle called entrainment, meaning the ability of two oscillating objects to come into synchronization. The music is like a "sound mirror" that, at first, reflects your current pain, and in the end, reflects the release and comfort you desire. Physically and/or emotionally, you transform along with the music.

You may not be familiar with the term entrainment but you likely will recognize the principle. Entrainment was first observed in the 17th century by Dutch scientist Christian Huygens. While working on the design of the pendulum clock, Huygens found that when he placed two clocks on a wall near each other and swung the pendulums at different speeds, they would eventually end up swinging at the same speed. This is due to their mutual influence on one another.

The classic example of entrainment shows individual pulsing heart muscle cells in a Petri dish. When they are brought close together, they begin pulsing in synchrony. Another example is women who live in the same household and often find that their menstrual cycles eventually coincide. The principle of entrainment is universal. It appears in chemistry, pharmacology, biology, medicine, psychology, sociology, astronomy, architecture, and of course, music.

MUSICAL ENTRAINMENT

Have you ever cried when you heard a certain musical composition or song? That is musical entrainment in process! The music had an influence on you, and you reacted on an emotional or a physical level. Certain sounds in specific sequence can help take the listener from one place to another.

What is it about music that generates this interesting response? Every parameter of music can have an entrainment effect, including tempo, rhythm, dynamics, pitch, harmony, articulation, and phrasing. The musical tempo and rhythms can become faster or slower, having an effect on the rhythms of your mind and body, including your heart rate. The dynamics can become softer or louder as the cells of your body feel caressed or released. The pitches and harmonies can become lower or higher as your emotions span a parallel range. The articulation and phrasing can become longer or shorter as your thoughts alternate between daydream and focus. Any one of these parameters can trigger a musical entrainment effect in the listener. *Music to Ease Chronic Pain* incorporates *all* of these parameters for the most powerful entrainment response possible. The result is a highly specialized music-healing experience that has the potential to:

- Resonate with the listener's feelings.

- Transform negativity into positivity.

- Promote a state of liveliness or serenity.

PAIN HAS A MEMORY

In ancient times, it would not have been considered strange to use sound for healing, but today it is not what people think of first when they are looking for pain relief. This is because human beings have changed over the eons. We now assume that only someone or something else has the power to heal. The *Holy Bible* states "Physician, heal yourself!" (Luke 4:23). Over time, this came to be known as: "Patient, heal thyself!" Even so, in these modern times, we seem to have collectively handed over the responsibility for our health to the medical community. In reality, it is not a black-and-white situation. Although we ultimately do heal ourselves, we do need help—guidance, medicine, therapies, and catalysts that initiate this road to recovery. *Music to Ease Chronic Pain* is such a catalyst. It triggers reactions within the listener that can initiate the body's own healing reflex. This music provides an innovative approach to relaxation, self-reflection, and acoustic resonance and can be a wonderful complement to your pain-release efforts.

Music has the distinct quality of being able to touch both the emotional and the physical parts of our being. Each person will respond differently to this music. Some people will experience more of an emotional response, and others will experience more of a physical response. It has been shown that there is a "mind-body link" between the emotional and physical. In fact, a whole specialization of medicine has evolved called *psychoneuroimmunology*, which shows there is an interconnection between psychology and neurology and their effect on the immune system. This means that certain emotional states are associated with certain physical conditions. If the emotional pain is reduced, it can indirectly help alleviate the physical condition. Similarly, if the physical pain is relieved, it can indirectly help the emotional state.

Different emotions are linked to various parts of the body. We tend to store these emotions physically in these parts of the body. This is called "cellular memory." We create cellular memory as a type of protection from feeling hurt or anger. When we finally let go of the old pain or anger, the current pain has nothing to cling to, and it too can be released. There are many methods of releasing this cellular memory. Music is one of the best ways because its vibration can permeate every cell of your body and help to unleash the stored block or pain.

Be patient, give it time and relax. Your trust in the music will offer the best results.

HOW THIS MUSIC WAS CREATED

I have been using my advanced music training and intuitive awareness to create music for transformation since 1982. First of all, let me say that I do not believe that there is any one definitive sound that could represent an individual's specific pain. There are too many variables, as the energy of our beings is constantly in flux. I believe, however, that what I've created can target the condition of pain in general, hopefully inclusive of most people's specific pain-related issues.

My process is actually uncomplicated. I use my intuition. I am aware that certain frequencies of music will resonate in different parts of the body and that certain rhythms can stimulate or relax systems in the body, like the beating of the heart, but the actual process that I use is to trust my intuition. Some people may call this "music channeling." In a way, I "tune in" to the condition and seek my highest awareness to create the best music to help a condition. In this music, it is pain.

My perception is mostly tactile, and sometimes auditory. I literally feel my hands on the piano keyboard being guided to their own choreography. This occurs until they are guided to stop and this becomes the end of the piece. My biggest challenge is to allow what I receive, and not try to interfere and alter a sound that I know will be dissonant.

There is no hypnosis, affirmations, subliminal messages, or guided imagery embedded in the music. The music is acoustic piano solo—nothing more.

PERSONAL STORIES

- In 1986, I was invited to present my paper, "Music for Pain Reduction," at the International Symposium of Music Medicine in Lüdenscheid, Germany. At the conference, I also offered to give a live demonstration to chronic-pain patients and then interview them afterward. I played the piano for four people from the local hospital who were in chronic pain. The conference attendees from around the world were watching and were quite skeptical. After I played, we had some amazing responses. One woman felt such relief from her back pain that she was crying.

- Another time, I did a live demonstration in California at a conference of health practitioners attending a bereavement seminar. One of the men came up to me afterward and told me that he had a very noticeable tingling in his arm exactly where he had had an injury from a car accident 20 years prior. This made sense to me immediately. I explained to him that the music was able to go deep into the cellular memory of the injury and his response was the tingling.

Over the years, I've had wonderful feedback from people from all over the world who've used my music to help their pain, including TMJ, back pain, tension headaches, and migraines.

Because I use my intuition to create my healing music, it often disappoints those people who are looking for some type of formula that can be logically explained. All I can say is that my ability to connect with a medical issue and create music for it has been fairly accurate. This ability has evolved over many years. I've done many personalized "Sound Portraits" of people, meaning I can put their true being to music, even if I don't know them well. One time I was doing some Sound Portraits in a group setting of strangers. One woman was chosen and I did not ask anything about her. I started playing this country western-sounding music. After I stopped, she was stunned and couldn't believe that I "got" her. She told me that she owns seven horses.

Guided Imagery:
A Mind/Body Experience

Judy Nelson

• • • • • • • • • • •

Guided imagery is a healing journey into your mind and body. It is an alternative therapy in which you use your mind's eye to visualize positive changes taking place in your body and in your thoughts and feelings.

Anyone who has ever daydreamed and can recall happy memories can benefit from guided imagery. In fact, if you close your eyes and concentrate on a specific image—whether it be a pretty scene or an image of your pain—you can master guided imagery. It may take a few tries to get a feel for it. At first, all you may be able to think about is what you are doing and how you are doing it. Eventually, without really being aware of it, you will naturally start to follow along. Suddenly you'll realize, "I got it!"

PICTURE OF PAIN

The guided imagery created for *Ease Chronic Pain* is designed to help you develop the power of your mind over your body by focusing on your thoughts. The words will help you paint a picture of your pain in your mind, then visualize it as images, light, color, and energy moving throughout and then out of your body. You will feel totally relaxed. The exercise will help you release tension and stress, and experience reduced pain or even a pain-free state. As you experience the imagery repeatedly over time, you may gradually deepen your ability to use visualizations to achieve more voluntary control over your pain.

Guided imagery is a healing art that has been used by alternative practitioners for hundreds of years. It is experiencing a rebirth and is now embraced by mainstream medicine and practiced in medical centers throughout the United States to help enhance the healing process. We have researchers and their scientific studies to thank for that because they have been able to prove why and how well it works.

HOW IT DE-STRESSES

Studies show that guided imagery has the ability to boost the immune system and promote healing. It has direct influence over the autonomic nervous system, which controls involuntary responses such as breathing and the beating of your heart. Guided imagery creates a state of relaxation, which automatically releases the stress that aggravates your pain. Studies have found it to be effective in reducing a number of chronic pain conditions, including lower back pain, tension headaches, migraines, and pain from conditions such as cancer, arthritis, and fibromyalgia.

- For example, studies at the Fred Hutchinson Cancer Center in Seattle showed significant relief of cancer pain when patients received a combination of guided imagery and relaxation techniques. In several studies using guided imagery for the treatment of headaches, participants experienced less intensity, duration of headaches, and/or increased ability to cope with them.

- Guided imagery has been found to be an effective treatment for stress associated with chronic pain. In several studies, guided imagery proved to help decrease the body's fight-or-flight response by helping people remain calm and feel less stressed. These studies revealed that people who practiced guided imagery and relaxation on their own achieved the greatest health benefits.

PRACTICE, PRACTICE

For all these reasons and more, the guided imagery for *Ease Chronic Pain* is presented as a complement to your pain-management plan. Allow yourself to experience the visualization at least once daily for 30 days. After that, the images will be so familiar to you that you will be able to walk yourself through them as needed throughout your day to release pain. Always use it in a quiet, peaceful setting and never when you have to put your concentration elsewhere, such as driving a car!

The script of what you will hear on the CD can be found on page 84. It is not necessary to read it before listening to the CD. It is totally your choice. You might prefer to listen to it first, then review it if you feel it will help you understand the process better. It is not intended or advised, however, to read it along with listening to the CD because you won't be able to get fully involved in the exercise. So, experiment—and enjoy.

Metaphysics and Music

Judy Nelson

• • • • • • • • • • •

SOUND HEALING HISTORY

During Renaissance times, the use of music in medicine continued to blossom. The theories of the ancient Greeks served as a foundation for music as a means of achieving physical harmony and balance. Renaissance music theorists paired four musical modes popular at the time with four musical elements (soprano, alto, tenor, and bass). These were linked to four bodily humors: choleric (related to the liver), sanguine (related to the heart), phlegmatic (related to the brain), and melancholic (related to the spleen).

Music was used in the treatment of these organs as well as pain, gout, sciatica, vermin bites, alcoholism, and mental disorders. Music was seen to evoke or ease particular emotions and was used in the treatment of depression and hysteria. Music was thought to promote a healthy immune system and increase resistance to disease, which was of vital importance in times of plague.

The field of quantum physics tells us that everything is made of energy. Even solid objects are made of energy, the components of which are actually in constant motion.

On the guided imagery track of the CD, you are introduced to a type of energy described as an electrical field that extends about a foot out from the body. According to the science of metaphysics, this energy field around us can hold our emotions and experiences. I have experienced this awareness of memories and emotions in the body many times. When I underwent deep-tissue body massage, the therapist pressed deeply on either side of my spine, and memories and emotions regarding my family arguing during my childhood surfaced in my mind. When he pressed on another area of my back, I reexperienced intense heartache from a romantic relationship that ended nearly twenty years ago. When he worked on my ankle, which had been strained several times over the years, I felt a deep grief being released over the death of my father fourteen years earlier.

ENERGY AT WORK

Metaphysicists believe that the body and energy field also hold trauma from past lives, and that this can be a major source of ill health and lack of balance in a person's life. They also believe that the body has highly charged energy centers, called chakras, at places where many nerve pathways intersect. Chakra is a Sanskrit word meaning "wheel that spins." Chakras are round disks of energy spinning inside the body. They function to receive, store, or release energy in the form of emotions, memories, or beliefs. Since chakras are in the body, their energy affects the body. Therefore, by cleaning and balancing a chakra you can help heal the part of the body that the chakra targets.

Certain types of music can stimulate specific chakras due to the lyrics, style, or intent of the composer. Here are some examples. If it doesn't feel right, go with what works for you.

First chakra (Physical). At the base of the spine.
Governs physical health as well as our physical experience in the world.
Traditional ethnic music, country and western, rap, big band.

Second chakra (Emotional). Just below the belly button.
Governs emotional health in regard to close relationships, as well as creativity and sensuality.
Gospel, R&B, blues.

Third chakra (Personal Power). The stomach.
Governs sense of personal power and ability to experience life, and reacts with balance and appropriate boundaries.
Rock, pop, metal.

Fourth chakra (Love for Self). Center of the chest.
Governs sense of self-love and love for the world.
Folk music, social consciousness songs, and world music.

Fifth chakra (Communication). The throat.
Governs inner voice and communication with others.
Opera, rap, musical theater, cabaret.

Sixth chakra (Intuition). Middle of the forehead.
Governs intuition.
New Age, wave, chanting, drumming.

Seventh chakra (Connection). The top of the head.
Governs personal control of life.
Jazz, classical, movie soundtracks, trance, minimalist, wave.

These three excercises are designed to help you relate to music on a metaphysical level.

Exercise 1

Music can help stimulate the energy in one or more chakras. If an area of your body is in pain, perhaps the chakra in that area is also out of balance. Try listening to music chosen by applying the "iso" principle—that is, music that reflects what you are feeling, then changes to music that shifts you to a healthier state of being. See if it stimulates a release of pain, stress, emotion, or excess energy in the area that is bothering you.

Choose a chakra in an area where you feel pain. Choose two musical pieces, with or without words. One should express your pain, and the other should express how you would like to feel. Close your eyes. Listen to the first selection and let it wash over you with its sound and meaning. Don't worry if it deepens your pain. Be aware of your pain, but start to take a step back from it and observe it as being governed by the chakra in that area.

When the first piece ends, pause, and visualize that chakra opening up and getting ready to release the pain. Then play the second piece, and imagine that the musical tones are actually entering the chakra through the back of your body, and pushing your pain out through the front of your body. As the pain is released, let the musical tones gently dance and swirl inside the chakra, filling it with a healing sound vibration that "tunes up" your chakra.

When the second piece ends, keep your eyes closed for another moment, and feel the power of music. Then take some time to write your experience in the journal beginning on page 64. Acknowledge all feelings that came up, as they are your body's way of speaking to you. If uncomfortable feelings arose, note them and brainstorm healthy, constructive ways to address these feelings.

Exercise 2

Go through your music collection and find a piece of music that makes you feel wonderfully alive. It can be long or short; just make sure that it makes you feel good. This music is a whole-body, whole-chakra balancer for you. Find a place to listen where you can feel free to move your body any way you want, hum, or sing along.

As you play the piece, allow yourself to participate by moving your body or using your voice. Let the music move through all of your chakras and your whole body.

After listening, write down three positive things the music made you feel. Use the same piece daily, until you feel ready for a different selection.

Exercise 3

Find a style of music that you would not typically listen to. As you listen to this musical style, observe how it makes you feel physically, emotionally, and even spiritually. Write your observations in your journal. If you enjoyed the music, you may want to expand your experience by attending a live concert of this type of music. The calendar section of your local newspaper is a great place to find out about musical events in your area. Use the journal to compare how recorded versus live music affects you. If you did not enjoy the music, try this exercise with other styles of music. You will begin to discover new music that provides a healing experience for you.

Other Self-Help Options

Howard Richman

• • • • • • • • • • •

SOUND HEALING HISTORY

Music continued to be used medicinally during the Baroque era. Physicians explored the psychological and neurological effects of music in a more systematic way, using scientific methods of observation to provide a factual basis for its healing effects. This scientific approach reinforced the belief that music had the power to affect body, mind, and emotions and supported the continued use of music for healing purposes. In the early 18th century royalty continued the practice of music as therapy, as is seen in the court of King Philip V of Spain. King Philip suffered from a depression so deep that the queen employed a famous Italian singer named Farinelli to sing to him every night to lift his spirits. References to the healing essence of music can be seen in the writings of Shakespeare and others of this time. The use of music as medicine was an accepted practice of the time.

Many people with chronic pain seek relief by trying different alternative therapies as a complement to traditional treatments. Though our expertise is in music healing and guided imagery, we are certainly aware, through our own experiences, that people with pain investigate many options. Listed here are those we think deserve mentioning. If any of these interest you, do your own research and discuss it with your pain-management provider. Do not change your pain-management program without the consent of your doctor.

Sometimes your pain is caused by an action you do every day, or by something that you wear, like a wallet in your back pocket. It requires some sleuthing but it can be a great relief to discover something very simple that has been causing so much pain.

For example, many people who wear bifocals tend to cock their necks upward when they look at a computer screen in order to see through their lower lens. After doing this for eight hours a day, it can cause quite a pain in the neck. Because I teach piano, I am aware of ergonomic obstacles such as this, but it is not obvious to most people. The solution here might be a special pair of glasses made with a slightly weaker prescription ("intermediate range"). The computer is usually slightly farther away than normal reading distance, does not require a full reading lens correction, and thus should not be limited by the lower lens of a bifocal.

Another source of pain is carpal tunnel syndrome or other repetitive-motion disorders. In some cases, there may be a physiological issue, but in most cases, the pain is caused by misuse or overuse. The book *Pain-Free Typing Technique* (Sound Feeling Publishing), outlines specific things you can do to prevent and reverse this type of pain. The most important thing to do is to observe if there is a bend anywhere between the hand, wrist, and arm. Usually the problem stems from the hand being bent at the wrist while the fingers are doing a task. This causes great friction and irritation, which over time can lead to pain. Adjust the height of your chair, the distance, and the angle of your arm until you get your lower arm, wrist, and hand in a straight line.

Hip or lower-back pain is often caused by something very common such the wallet in the back pocket mentioned earlier. Not only does this cause a rotation of the hip joint in an unnatural way, but it also throws your body off balance when you are sitting. Think about this: After years and years of sitting with one side of your body a half-inch higher than the other side, do you really wonder why you have hip pain?

There may be something that is not so obvious in relation to your personal pain that, when removed, will have a profound effect. You may not be able to determine what it is because your habits are ingrained and you are unaware of the things you do that result in pain. In this case, have someone observe you doing daily tasks and see if they notice anything that could be causing or aggravating your problem.

DIET

Do you ever notice that your pain flares up or perhaps subsides after eating certain foods? Certain painful conditions are directly related to the food you eat.

For example, gout, which causes severe pain, is the result of an accumulation of uric acid, usually in the big toe. It is caused by eating a diet rich in purines, which are found in such foods as seafood and organ meats. Your doctor can help guide you to pain relief through diet and medication.

A common type of chronic pain is headaches. Until the age of 18, I had migraine-type headaches almost every single day. I did all kinds of research in an effort to find the cause. The one thing that finally had the most impact was eliminating margarine and hydrogenated vegetable oil from my diet.

It turns out that this type of fat, which is so prevalent in many packaged foods, can clog the microcapillaries in the brain.

Another specific food-related illness is celiac disease, which is caused by the inability to properly digest wheat and foods that contain gluten. It causes severe digestive distress.

Some other painful conditions may be related to diet but are not as easy to pinpoint. There are a variety of foods, for example, that, over time, can aggravate rheumatoid arthritis. Among the suspects are milk, red meat, sugar, citrus, eggplant, tomatoes, potatoes, and salt.

In general, nutritionists suggest that following a healthy diet low in fat and free of processed foods can help people tolerate pain better because it helps put them in an otherwise state of good health. You may want to consider talking to a nutritionist to address your specific issues. Check the Internet or your local health organizations to find a qualified nutritionist who specializes in pain management.

CHIROPRACTIC

Traditional medicine primarily treats the symptoms, whereas chiropractic attempts to treat the underlying cause of the problem. A chiropractor detects misalignments and corrects them through adjustments that move bones and spinal discs back into position. A chiropractor will often recommend specific exercises to strengthen muscle groups around the afflicted area so that the adjustment will "hold." Chiropractic is recognized by the American Medical Association and is covered by Medicare and most insurance carriers.

Most people assume that a chiropractor is only for back pain, but many types of pain can be helped by a chiropractor. When you are watering your plants with a hose and the hose gets a kink in it, the water slows to a trickle until you unkink it. Well, the same is true for the nerves that go to various parts of your body. Each vertebra of your spinal column has nerves that connect to specific organs and limbs. If the spine is out of alignment, this could impinge on the neural flow and compromise the correct functioning of that part of the body, or even create pain.

The best source for finding a good chiropractor is to get a recommendation from someone you trust. Also, the American Chiropractic Association (www.acatoday.com) has a referral list of qualified chiropractors.

DRINKING WATER

Most people with chronic pain tend to be dehydrated. According to Fereydoon Batmanghelidj, M.D., author of *Water for Health, for Healing, for Life*, the body uses pain as an emergency call for water. It can come in the form of heartburn, joint pain, back pain, migraine headaches, colitis pain, fibromyalgia pain, even angina pain, says Dr. Batmanghelidj. When there isn't enough fluid to be evenly distributed throughout the body, certain parts of the body have trouble eliminating toxins. As toxic waste builds up, the nerve endings in that area register the chemical environmental change with the brain. The brain translates this information for the conscious mind in the form of pain.

Keep in mind that coffee, soft drinks, and alcohol tend to dehydrate cells and are not a substitute for water. In fact, caffeine and alcohol act as diuretics. Some nutritionists recommend that every 6 ounces of caffeine or alcohol consumed should be supplemented with 10 to 12 ounces of water.

What kind of water is best? Purified, bottled, reverse-osmosis, distilled, tap, spring? Yikes—the choices could drive you crazy! The one thing that most health practitioners tend to agree on is that we should drink nonchlorinated water.

One folk remedy for arthritis is drinking distilled water because it contains no minerals. Paul C. Bragg, N.D., Ph.D., in his book, *Water: The Shocking Truth That Can Save Your Life*, advocates drinking distilled water for health, and particularly for arthritis. According to Dr. Bragg, distilled water binds with minerals that can clog joints and excretes them through the urine. There is some controversy on how long one should drink distilled water. Some people believe that at some point, the distilled water begins to remove minerals necessary for health. Others believe that it is nature's water (rain water is distilled) and that it can be consumed indefinitely. Regardless, you should try this only with the consent and supervision of your doctor.

SUPPLEMENTS

There are many natural nutritional and herbal supplements on the market purported to help alleviate pain. Before trying any, make sure to do your homework. Go to a health-food store and talk to a qualified person who can help you. Keep in mind that just because a substance is natural does not mean that it is automatically safe. Also, what works for one type of pain may not work for another.

For example, herbs known to help relieve headache are not necessarily good for skin irritation or stomach or foot pain. It is to your advantage to do your own research and talk to your pain-management practitioner to help find what is best for you. If you and your practitioner decide a supplement is worth trying, keep in mind that more is not better. Exceeding recommended dosages can be dangerous. Some supplements do not mix with certain medications. You should consult with your doctor and pharmacist about everything you are taking, both natural and pharmaceutical, before supplementing. Here are just a few of the supplements that may help quell various types of pain.

Aloe Vera. Burns, hemorrhoids, infection, rash, skin problems, sunburn.

Chamomile. Bunions, carpal tunnel syndrome, gum disease, heartburn, indigestion, infections, insect bites, ulcers.

Choline. Nervous system disorders.

Evening Primrose Oil. Headache, menstrual cramps, skin problems.

Horsetail. Gout, kidney stones, joint pain.

Peppermint. Backache, earache, fever, gallstones, gum disease, headache, heartburn, indigestion, sinusitis.

Valerian Root. Intestinal spasms, stress.

Vitamin B Complex. Arthritis, carpal tunnel syndrome, kidney stones, mouth sores, stress.

Vitamin C. Arteriosclerosis, arthritis, colds, gum disease, stress, wounds.

White Willow Bark. Arthritis, backache, carpal tunnel syndrome, colds, earache, gout, headache, sciatica, tendonitis, toothache.

Wintergreen Oil. Backache, earache, sore throat.

PSYCHOTHERAPY

It is not unheard of for an unhealed, unrelated emotional issue to crop up years later as pain in a specific part of the body. For many people, holding in feelings is habitual. This creates a body armor built up over time that can result in disease and pain. This takes place in what is called the "cellular memory."

I've noticed that when I have a difficult decision to make, it can give me a headache. I've also noticed that if I want to say something to someone but do not, I often get a sore throat. I've observed friends who regret not having had a baby deal with perpetual "stomach" pains. Louise Hay, in her book, *Heal Your Body*, shows how feeling unsupported can result in lower back pain.

If you think that an emotional experience could be aggravating your pain or be the root of your pain, you may want to consider short-term counseling. It could be a catalyst in freeing emotionally induced physical pain.

BREATHING

Obviously, you are breathing—but are you breathing properly? Pain can cause people to breathe less deeply. This happens for many reasons. The saying "It only hurts when I laugh" actually is true for many types of pain, and it correlates to breathing.

Deep breathing requires movement within the body, which can aggravate certain types of pain. As a result, you unconsciously suppress your natural way of breathing.

A state of anticipation or worry can cause shallow breathing. If you are worrying about your pain returning, it's like the dreaded wait for the other shoe to drop. This type of anxiety can cause a cycle of pain and worry.

Deep breathing, on the other hand, is good for you on several levels. It supplies your organs with vitally needed oxygen. Organs that are functioning optimally can help reduce the pain cycle.

Breathing deeply also is one of the best means to help get rid of waste products and toxins from your cells. Metabolic toxic buildup in your system is one of the things that causes the perception of pain in the first place. Deep breathing also helps to bring hidden emotions to the surface. If there are any hidden emotions that are anchored to your pain—the mind/body connection—it is to your advantage to let it show itself. The guided imagery in this program may be able to help you recognize these emotions. There are many breathing techniques that can help lead to wellness. Do a little research. You might want to investigate the techniques called Pranayama, and Rebirthing or Breathwork. Just having the willpower, however, to remember to breath deeply may be all you need to get the benefits.

VISUALIZATIONS AND AFFIRMATIONS

It is possible to direct your thoughts to your areas of pain to help effect a change. Our subconscious mind is kind of like the master projector of our lives. What we believe deeply or hold true will manifest itself. Some people believe that the reason we have pain in our lives is that for some reason, however inadvertently, we have created it or attracted it to ourselves.

A visualization is a positive image that you consciously see in your mind, and an affirmation is a positive statement that you say outwardly or inwardly. The guided imagery in this program makes use of both visualizations and affirmations. In addition to this wonderful tool, you may want to create some customized visualizations or affirmations to help you with your specific pain situation.

Create visualizations and affirmations in current time using images and positive words. This means that you should see what you want as if it has already occurred. Say them and see them in your mind's eye with a deep feeling of truth on a regular basis. This is the way to reprogram your subconscious mind. When this happens, your outer reality will change. Here are some examples:

- **Back pain:** *"My back is flexible and strong!"*

- **Foot pain:** *"My feet take me wherever I want to go!"*

- **Hand pain in a pianist:** *"I can play the piano easily and freely."*

- **Headache:** *"My head is clear and relaxed."*

- **Hip pain:** *"I can move my hips with ease."*

ELECTROMAGNETIC POLLUTION

Healthy cells, according to Nobel prize-winner Otto Warburg, have cell voltages of 70 to 90 millivolts. Due to the constant stresses of modern life and a toxic environment, cell voltage tends to drop as we age or get sick. As the voltage drops, the cell is unable to maintain a healthy environment. If the electrical charge of a cell drops to 50, a person may experience chronic fatigue. If the voltage drops to 15, the cell often can be cancerous.*

To us, it seems logical to assume that the proximity of various electrical devices can have an influence on cellular electricity within the body, and there is growing evidence to support this. Different voltages can disrupt the subtle millivoltages that our cells require. When the cells are not functioning optimally, it can cause not only pain but also illness. There are two excellent books on this subject: *Cross Currents* by Robert O. Becker, M.D. (Jeremy P. Tarcher, 1990) and *Bioelectromagnetic Healing* by Thomas Valone (Integrity Research Institute, 2000).

Recording engineers know that if they run an audio cable parallel to an AC (household alternating current) power cable, a hum will result in the audio cable. However, if the wires cross in a perpendicular fashion, there will be no hum. If you can alter the influence that a power cord can have on an audio cable, a similar effect could occur in the body.

Be aware of things you might do in your own home to minimize or to alter the influence of this electromagnetic "pollution." For example, simply rotating the head of your bed to a different direction or moving it away from the wall

---

* Warburg, Otto. "On the Origin of Cancer Cells," *Science*, Vol. 123 (1956): 309.

can have a profound effect on certain types of pain. This is because the wiring inside the walls may be too close to your head when you sleep, disrupting your cellular millivoltages.

EXERCISE AND PHYSICAL THERAPY

When it comes to pain, exercise seems counter intuitive. The last thing you want to do is move your body when you are in pain, but it may be the best thing. When you have pain, however, it is crucial that you do not embark on an exercise program by yourself or you could do more damage. Always consult with a professional physical therapist or a pain-management specialist or a trainer who knows about pain.

Some physical therapies are passive in nature. They are used to increase blood flow to the afflicted area, which stimulates healing. The most common passive techniques are heat and ice-pack alternations, TENS (Transcutaneous Electrical Nerve Stimulation) units, massage, and ultrasound devices. Active physical therapy involves exercises, including stretching and strengthening and aerobic exercises.

Assuming you have the go-ahead and the guidance from your pain-management specialist, the following suggestions will help make your exercise program more effective.

- **Customized exercises.** Let's say that you recognize the benefits of aerobic exercise. If you are prone to knee pain, jumping may not be a good idea. You could, however, sit on the trampoline and gently bounce to get an aerobic workout, and it will indirectly help your painful areas without subjecting them to stress.

- **Aquatic Therapy.** There are wonderful exercises that you can do in a swimming pool with special equipment. The anti gravity effect of being in the water will give you the benefit of the exercise without endangering the afflicted area. Aquatic therapy requires the supervision of a trained pain-management specialist.

- **Cool-downs.** The right kind of exercise can help heal pain, temporarily, but without a proper cool-down, the pain could become even worse. Exercise creates more flow in the body and flow is good—blood flow, oxygen flow, lymph flow, blocked-energy flow. A lot of pain is physically caused by a buildup of lactic acid in the tissue. The problem is that if you exercise and then stop suddenly, more lactic acid builds up than if you also do a proper cool-down. For example, if you run a mile and then just stop, your legs will hurt the next day. But if you walk for another third of a mile to cool down, you will force the lactic acid to continue circulating and gradually leave the body.

Create Your Own Healing Music

Howard Richman

• • • • • • • • • • •

SOUND HEALING HISTORY

Scientific advances of the 19th century gave physicians the ability to precisely measure physiological responses to music. Music's effect on blood pressure, heart rate, digestion, and volume and rate of respiration were studied. Musicians and scientists of the time, such as the famous composer Hector Berlioz *(Symphonie fantastique)*, researched and reported music's effects on relieving stress and curing illness. Magazine articles started surfacing in the United States documenting the effectiveness of music in treating depression and other maladies. In 1806, Samuel Matthews noted the use of music to counteract pain in his dissertation, On the Effects of Music in Curing and Palliative Diseases. The use of music to treat psychological disorders increased as the body of evidence grew documenting music's positive effects on the psyche. By the late 19th century, the therapeutic use of music expanded into schools for the deaf, blind, and handicapped, as well as hospitals and institutions in the United States and England.

You can create your own healing music recording, and you don't even have to play a musical instrument to do it. All you have to do is make your own cassette, CD, or digital song list by sequencing existing compositions together following the principle of entrainment that was used in composing *Music to Ease Chronic Pain.*

USE EXISTING MUSIC IN A NEW WAY

First choose music that totally matches your current mood rather than the mood you wish to acquire. I like to use depression as an example because it is an easy concept to follow. Select a composition that to you represents depression in its most extreme form. Follow this with one that is only mildly depressing. Then select a neutral composition, and end with a composition that is clearly uplifting and motivating.

Apply the same idea to your pain. Be careful not to do the typical thing, which is to play some very, very, soothing music right at the start. This might be nice to hear, but it will likely not have a healing effect, because it will not mirror your current condition. In fact, if you play something that is so different than how you currently feel, it could have the effect of increasing your pain! This is because of the disparity between what you hear and how you feel.

Listening to music in a sequence like this allows your current stress or pain level or mood to be first honored and then gradually transformed. The *Music to Ease Chronic Pain* on the CD uses this sequencing technique but in a very advanced way.

COMPOSING ORIGINAL MUSIC

If you play an instrument, you could try composing your own original music following the same technique. Once you understand the concept, and with some experimentation, you may be very effective in personalizing this modality. You can do this intuitively or you can do it intellectually. Both methods have value. Get your tape-recorder, CD burner, or midi-sequencer ready!

The intuitive method is appropriate if you already are aware of your connection to your intuition or "higher self." You can ask your higher self (or God, or your spirit guides, depending on your belief system) to guide you in creating the perfect music that will be helpful to release your pain. Really wait and see if something arises from within that is different than the normal way that you would play your instrument. This is basically a type of improvisation but it would be considered nonmental or "free" improvisation.

The intellectual way of creating a customized piece of healing music is equally valid. Your music training tells you that certain harmonies are dissonant and others are consonant. Certain rhythms evoke stress and others evoke a sense of relaxation. Use your musical knowledge to create sounds that give your pain a chance to "speak." Then, very gradually transition this music into something that would be identified with a lack of pain.

Listen to your creation repeatedly and notice if the fact that you created it yourself has a distinct benefit to you in helping to lessen or remove your pain.

Making your own healing music can be very rewarding. There is evidence that creating your own music is good for your health. A study at Willamette University in Salem, Oregon investigated the effects of making music (active music) and listening to music (passive music) on 33 undergraduate students. They were divided into three groups: One group listened to live music; one group sang and played percussion instruments; and one group was not exposed to any type of music at all. When tested, the students who sang and played music exhibited a marked increase in immune-boosting chemicals over both other groups.

This, of course, is no surprise to us. If you have been contemplating taking music lessons or joining a choir, this may be the time to do it for your health and wellness.

About Music Therapy

In the early to mid-20th century, experiments continued to demonstrate the various effects of music on emotions and physiology. Psychologists became increasingly interested in music's effects on mood and state of mind. Music began to be used in the operating room as an aid to anesthesia, and in the recovery room for pain management for patients after operations.

The music and guided imagery in this program were specially created to inspire relaxation, release pain, and offer you the potential to experience the healing effects of these two techniques in the comfort of your own home.

Although the practices outlined here will have a therapeutic effect, it is not truly music therapy. Music therapy by definition requires the presence of a certified and trained music therapist during the music activity, and that the therapist continually design the activity to address the specific needs of the patient. With this program, you are accessing the potential benefits of listening to healing music and guided imagery on your own.

The Biomedical Theory of Music Therapy suggests in part that music can produce a desired response in the central nervous system. Even though you may not be working with a music therapist directly, it is possible to experience positive effects by listening to music on your own. The way the auditory system develops may explain why humans are highly responsive to music.

During pregnancy, the ear first appears at approximately 22 days' gestation. Studies show that in the first trimester, a fetus can perceive sound. This is quite early in your "existence." Actual hearing begins at 25 weeks. By the 5th to 7th month, sound is being transmitted to the brain where it can be perceived and remembered.

In studies where music was played to the fetus through headphones placed on the mother's abdomen, fetal heart-rate changes were seen consistently. This early development of hearing structures indicates that sound may be stimulating the fetal brain and helping to form cognitive structures that continue to develop after birth. During the entire time the fetus can hear and process sound, it is experiencing the steady, rhythmic pulse of the mother's heartbeat. This may explain why even young babies move their bodies instinctively when they hear rhythmic music.

THE BASIS OF MUSIC THERAPY

Music therapy blends the knowledge of sound vibration with the aesthetics of art for the purposes of achieving an improved state of health. A basic definition of music therapy is that it is the prescribed use of music by a trained specialist for the therapeutic benefit of the client. There are five elements to this definition:

- Music is the main modality used in treatment during music therapy. Other modalities of expression may be present, such as talking, movement, imagery, or art, but music is the focus of the experience.

- Music is prescribed. In music therapy, the choice of musical styles, tempos, and orchestration is not random. Music is carefully selected by the trained specialist based on the iso principle. The iso principle advocates that the music therapist first use music that matches the mood and physiological state of the client, and then gradually change the music to alter the state of the client, with the aim of achieving improved mental, emotional, and/or physical health.

- Music is applied by a trained specialist. Since music evokes emotions and affects physiology and state of mind, it is essential that music therapy be conducted by a musician who has attained specialized skills. Music therapy training currently includes courses in anatomy, psychology, and special education, in addition to rigorous field work under experienced supervision. This training prepares the therapist to address the varied psychosocial needs of the client that arise during music therapy treatment.

- Music is applied for therapeutic benefit. Music activities in and of themselves may be just plain fun, but the true purpose of music therapy is to provide an experience through which the client may achieve improved physical, emotional, and/or psychological health.

- The client is the center of the music therapy process. All activities are intended, designed, and implemented for the client's needs.

This is why music therapy is not simply music sent home by the therapist for clients to listen to on their own. It is the relationship of trust that develops between the therapist and the client through the music experience that provides an environment for the iso principle to be applied.

THE HISTORY OF MUSIC THERAPY

The first courses in music therapy in the United States were offered in 1919 at Columbia University in New York by Margaret Anderton, who had used music to treat Canadian soldiers during World War I. In 1926, the National Association for Music in Hospitals was established to standardize the role and practice of musicians working in hospitals and institutions in the United States. The National Foundation for Music Therapy was established in 1941 by Harriet Seymour, who was an advocate of music therapy in helping injured veterans of World War II. As a result, music therapy programs began to spring up in hospitals throughout the United States.

In 1944, what is now Michigan University established the first curriculum to train music therapists. Programs were subsequently established at various colleges and universities throughout the United States and then throughout the world. The first music therapy organization was established in the United States in 1950, and is now known as the American Music Therapy Association.

Your Healing Journal

· · · · · · · · · · · ·

Healing music and guided imagery are healing arts, but they are also creative arts. They can inspire the listener in creative ways as well.

As you listen to the music and guided imagery on the *Ease Chronic Pain* CD, allow your creativity and insight to surface from the depths of your inner psyche, and use this journal to write down your thoughts and experiences as you progress through the program. It can be an empowering part of the healing process.

This journal is your special section for personal reflection. Use it to freely express your feelings about your pain. If you find the process difficult, use one of the following exercises for inspiration.

Exercise 1: My Reflections

After you listen to the CD, close your eyes for a moment to feel the power of the music, then take at least five minutes to sit down and write about your response to the music and/or guided imagery. Complete the following thoughts honestly and fully to allow your inner voice to communicate with your conscious mind through your writing:

- *I thought about . . .*

- *My body felt . . .*

- *My emotions felt . . .*

- *Now I am experiencing . . .*

- *With this knowledge about myself, I will use this experience in the following way to ease my chronic pain . . .*

Exercise 2: My Musical Style

Think of yourself as a musical style—classical, jazz, Top 40, and so on. What best expresses your personality? The style you choose is symbolic of your true essence. Answer the following questions and explain why that style reflects the real you:

- *How does this music reflect what is important to me in my life?*

- *Is my life in balance with these important aspects of my life?*

- *What is needed to enhance it or get me there?*

Perhaps you are a sentimental love song. This suggests that romance, love, and close relationships are important to you and support your health and healing. Consequently, if those relationships are out of balance in your life, this exercise clarifies and affirms an area of your life that you would like to improve.

If you are unclear about what type of music symbolizes you, just start writing about yourself in your journal. In time, your own inner wisdom about what makes you unique will be reflected in your journal.

Exercise 3: My Favorite Music

Studies show that listening to music you prefer can help boost your immune system and lift your mood. Harness that power and apply it in your life by creating a "My Favorite Music" program. Compile 45 minutes of your favorite songs or compositions, or purchase your favorite CD. Listen to it whenever the spirit moves you. When you grow tired of listening to it, make or buy a new one with completely different musical selections.

Keep all of your personal creations in a library of "My Favorite Music" and go back and listen to them periodically. Let your favorite music program guide you to a place of physical, mental, emotional, and spiritual healing. After you listen to one of your customized music programs, use your journal to record how the music inspired you, what it made you think about, and how it made you feel.

Notice what your psyche is communicating to you through your creative journal writing. The music may inspire messages from your wise inner voice to your conscious mind.

Life is the notes right underneath your fingers. All you have to do
is take time out to play the right notes.

RAY CHARLES

If you can walk, you can dance. If you can talk, you can sing.
ZIMBABWE PROVERB

Music washes away from the soul the dust of everyday life.
BERTHOLD AUERBACH

Music is the shorthand of emotion.
LEO TOLSTOY

If music be the food of love, play on.
WILLIAM SHAKESPEARE

Take a music-bath once or twice a week for a few seasons,
and you will find that it is to the soul what the water-bath is to the body.

OLIVER WENDELL HOLMES

Music melts all the separate parts of our bodies together.

ANAIS NIN

Music is the art which is most nigh to tears and memory.

OSCAR WILDE

Music hath charms to soothe the savage breast,
To soften rocks, or bend a knotted oak.

WILLIAM CONGREVE

The truest expression of a people is in its dances and its music.
AGNES DE MILLE

Music is the sole domain in which man realizes the present.
IGOR STRAVINSKY

In music the passions enjoy themselves.
FRIEDRICH NIETZSCHE

Music is a beautiful opiate . . .
HENRY MILLER

You are the music while the music lasts.
T. S. ELIOT

Music is moonlight in the gloomy night of life.
JEAN-PAUL RICHTER

Who hears music, feels his solitude peopled at once.
ROBERT BROWNING

Guided Imagery for Pain Release (CD Script)

Text of spoken words on CD track 3

Find a quiet place with a comfortable chair where you can relax free from distraction and interruptions. Dim the lights if you prefer. This is your time for meditation, imagery, and relaxation.

Sit comfortably in your chair. Take off your shoes. Place your feet flat on the floor, and gently rest your hands on top of your thighs, with your palms facing up.

Pain and discomfort will be released through your hands. Close your eyes, and take just a moment to relax.

Take a deep, slow breath. Inhale . . . and exhale. Another deep breath. Inhale . . . and exhale. And one more deep breath. Inhale . . . and exhale.

Feel your physical body sitting in the chair. Feel your feet flat on the floor. Be aware of your physical body.

You also have an energy body that is the same size and shape as your physical body, but it is made only of energy. It is right there with your physical body. Often, when you are in a state of physical discomfort, you may feel disoriented from your physical body, as if you're not all here. This is part of your energy body floating away. Now, image your energy body coming back to your physical body. Your energy body fits directly inside your physical body, just underneath your skin. Imagine your energy body standing in front you, with its back to you. Place your energy body inside your physical body by having your energy body sit directly into your physical body. Its feet fit inside your feet. Its hips fit inside your hips. Its shoulders fit inside your shoulders. And its head fits inside your head. Your energy body is now aligned perfectly inside your physical body, directly underneath your skin. Feel it. With your energy body aligned inside your physical body, you are ready to bring a sense of healing and wholeness to your entire self.

Now, you are going to anchor your energy body inside your physical body to give your physical body a sense of stability and support by creating a beam of energy that grounds your physical body into the earth. Be aware of your spine— specifically, the bottom of your spine, at the end of your tailbone. Imagine your spine not only as a physical part of your body but as an energy part of your body, too—energy that is generated by the nerves that travel up and down the spinal cord. This energy pathway is filled with the energy of life itself—so much so that you can imagine the bottom of your tailbone growing longer and extending down from the body like an energy beam of golden sunlight.

Image your tailbone extending this golden light down through the chair and beaming through the floor beneath your feet, effortlessly into the earth, like a root. Image this beam of golden light traveling deep into the soil of our rich and beautiful planet. Extend it until it connects with the very center of the earth. This is your grounding energy beam, and it extends from the end of your tailbone to the center of the earth. Image this extension of your spine as an organic, natural part of you that is strong and flexible, providing your body with a sense of support and stability, just as a plant is supported by being rooted deep into the earth. Your grounding beam of energy is making your physical body feel safe and secure as you engage in imagery to release your pain and create a change within yourself.

In our meditation, you are going to image golden sunlight all around you and through you. It is a gentle vibration that is healing, calming, and soothing.

Now, be aware of a golden point of light as it centers on your forehead. Focus your attention . . . your consciousness . . . your awareness . . . to that point of light in the center of your forehead. Now, move that golden point of light in your forehead back to the center of your brain—right between the left and right hemispheres.

Let the golden point of light fill your mind and your thoughts. Your entire brain is filled with golden sunlight. This is your centering point—your focus point. Feel your thoughts gently dissolve into pools of golden light, and let a sense of peace fill your awareness. Feel the stillness, the calm, slow vibration of your brain waves— slower . . . gently—to the level just before sleep.

You are now centered and grounded. Be aware of your feet planted solidly on the floor, offering your body an additional sense of support and stability.

Your body and your brain are amazing energy-makers. Your brain is a central processing center. It receives information from your body and processes it in order to make sense out of it. And then it sends signals out to the body, telling it how to feel, and how to respond. When your awareness is that golden point of light right between the hemispheres of your brain, you are in your body's true energy center. Through your breathing, imagery, and relaxation, you are able to send healing and comfort out from this center into all areas of the physical body. And since the body is wired to respond to your brain's messages, your body shifts to these images of relaxation and wellness.

Now, as you are focusing on your breathing, image a sky-blue energy entering your lungs, and moving into all the nerve pathways in your body, soothing and calming them. And exhale, feeling a release of tension. Slowly breathe in, sending sky-blue energy through every nerve pathway in the body. Exhale, and feel the release in these pathways as your pain, tension, and stress let go. Again, inhale. Bring the sky-blue energy into the lungs, and out through every nerve pathway in your body . . . exhale. Release pain . . . tension . . . stress. Inhale into your lungs . . . out the nerve pathways. Exhale . . . and release pain, tension, stress. You are bathing your nerve pathways in a healing and soothing sky-blue energy that calms and relaxes, and brings a sense of peace to the nervous system. If there are any emotions that are being held along the nerve pathways, the sky-blue energy engulfs them and pulls them out and releases them as you exhale. If you feel discomfort in any area of your body, direct the sky-blue energy there, and let it enter . . . and release the pain as you inhale and exhale. Inhale again, sending sky-blue energy to those points in your body that hold discomfort. Exhale . . . and let the sky-blue energy carry it out. Again, inhale . . . and exhale. Inhale again, allowing the sky-blue energy into every pore of your body. And exhale, releasing all your excess emotion, tension, and pain.

Now, shift color to a beautiful light green—the color of new leaves springing forth on a plant. Inhale, and pull the light green into your skin and muscles to regenerate your cells and bring growth and healing to every area of your body. Exhale, releasing emotions, tension, and pain. Breathe in again. Let it fill up your muscles with its life-giving energy. And exhale, releasing emotions, tension, and pain. Inhale. Feel the light green enter the skin and fill your muscles and cells. Exhale. Release all excess emotion, tension, and pain. And once again, light green filling up your skin and muscles. Exhale . . . and release.

Now, breathe in golden sunlight, filling up every cell in your bones, muscles, veins and arteries, nerve pathways, and skin. It is the most beautiful golden sunlight, breathe it in. Exhale, and release. Once again, breathe in the gold sunlight as if you are breathing into every single part of your body. The pores of your skin are absorbing it; your lungs are filled with it. Exhale, letting go of tension and pain. Release. One more time, breathe in gold light. Fill in every inch of your body— it's tingling and alive. Yet it is calm, peaceful, and centering. And exhale.

At this time, your breathing feels deep, calm, and relaxing. Image that the point of light in the center of your brain between your hemispheres is growing into a beautiful golden ball of sunlight—sunlight that is bathing all of your brain tissue. Calming . . . soothing . . . slowing your brain waves. . . . It is now activating your parasympathetic nervous system that allows you to return to a state of balance.

If you are still feeling any pain or discomfort in the body, imagine that you have an energy sponge, and place it right into that area of discomfort. Let the energy sponge soak up the pain or discomfort—as much as it possibly can. When the sponge is saturated, pull it out. Imagine that it is gently floating away from you. When the sponge is about 5 feet away, place a golden ball of sunlight under the sponge. Squeeze pain energy out of the sponge into the ball of light. The ball of light absorbs the pain. Then fling that ball of light into the sky, and let it transform back into the energy of life once again. You can insert that energy sponge into any area of the body as many times as you like. Let the sponge soak up the pain . . . pull the sponge out . . . and squeeze it into a golden ball of sunlight a few feet away from you. Send the ball of light out into the sky to become the energy of life. Again, insert the energy sponge, let the sponge soak up the pain . . . pull the sponge out . . . and squeeze it into a golden ball of sunlight a few feet away from you. Send the ball of light out into the sky to become the energy of life. You are done with the energy sponge for now. Place the sponge in a golden ball of sunlight, and send it out into the sky to again transform into the energy of life.

Now you are ready to fill yourself up with the most soothing and healing energy that exists. Imagine a radiant golden sun above your head, beaming with light. Gently feel the sun sink down into your face, filling it up with golden light. Bring the golden sun into your throat, filling it with the soothing golden light. Let the gold light gently move down your shoulders . . . down your arms . . . into your hands . . . and extend into each of your fingertips. Let the golden light come down into your chest and bathe your heart and lungs. Feel the golden light move down *your torso, filling your stomach. Let it move down into your hips, filling your intestines and internal organs with gentle, golden light. Move the light down your legs, filling your bones and muscles with light. Let the golden light move into your knees, and fill them up. Let the light move down through your calves and fill your ankles with pools of gold. The golden light moves into your feet, filling them up, all the way to the ends of your toes. Feel yourself filled with the divine essence of life itself, relaxing you, nurturing you.*

Take another deep breath—inhale . . . and exhale. You have been in an altered state of consciousness for a while, and now it is time to bring your focus back to the here and now. As you sit with your eyes closed, be aware of the chair beneath your body . . . the floor beneath your feet . . . and the sounds around you. Take three deep breaths. Nice and easy. One . . . two . . . three. . . . Breathe naturally. Bring your focus back to this time and place. Gently move your toes. Stretch your arms and legs. You are now ready to open your eyes, look around, and reorient yourself.

Congratulations! You have given yourself the gift of meditation and imagery. You have released the pain and replaced it with healing light. May it bring you a sense of peace, wholeness, and wellness.

References

Aldridge, D. *Music Therapy Research and Practice in Medicine: From Out of the Silence*. (London: Jessica Kingsley Publishers, Inc., 1996).

Balch, J. and Balch, P. *Prescription for Nutritional Healing: A Practical A-Z Reference to Drug-Free Remedies Using Vitamins, Minerals, Herbs and Food Supplements*. (Garden City Park, New York: Avery Publishing Group, 1990).

Bartlett, D.; Kaufman, D.; and Smeltekop, R. "The Effects of Music Listening and Perceived Sensory Experiences on the Immune System as Measured by Interleukin-1 and Cortisol," *Journal of Music Therapy*, Vol. 30, Issue 4 (1993): 194–209.

Bob, S. "Audioanalgesia in Podiatric Practice—A Preliminary Study," *Journal of American Podiatry Association*, 52 (1962): 503–504.

Boldt, S. "The Effects of Music Therapy on Motivation, Psychological Well-Being, Physical Comfort, and Exercise Endurance of Bone Marrow Transplant Patients," *Journal of Music Therapy*, Vol. *33*, Issue 3 (1996): 164-88.

Bonny, H. *Guided Imagery and Music Therapy: Past, Present and Future Implications*. (Baltimore: ICM Books, 1978).

Brown, C.; Chen, A.; and Dworkin, S. "Music in the Control of Human Pain," *Music Therapy*, Vol. 8, Issue 11 (1989): 47–60.

Cherry, H., and Pallin. I. "Music as a Supplement in Nitrous Oxide-Oxygen Anesthesia," *Anesthesiology*, 9 (1948): 391–99

Chesky, K., and Michel, D. "The Music Vibration Table (MVT): Developing a Technology and Conceptual Model for Pain Relief," *Music Therapy Perspectives*, 9 (1991): 32–38.

Chiles, Pila. *The Secrets and Mysteries of Hawaii: A Call to the Soul.* (Deerfield Beach, Florida: Health Communications, Inc., 1995).

Clark, M.; McCorkle, R.; and Williams, S. "Music Therapy-Assisted Labor and Delivery," *Journal of Music Therapy*, Volume 18, Issue 2 (1981): 88–109.

Colwell, C. "Music as a Distraction and Relaxation to Reduce Chronic Pain and Narcotic Ingestion: A Case Study," *Music Therapy Perspectives*, Vol. 15, Issue 1 (1997): 24–31.

Davis, W. and Thaut, M. "The Influence of Preferred Relaxing Music on Measures of State Anxiety, Relaxation, and Physiological Responses," *Journal of Music Therapy*, Vol. 26, Issue 4 (1989): 168–87.

Duke, J. *The Green Pharmacy: The Ultimate Compendium of Natural Remedies from the World's Foremost Authority on Healing Herbs*. (New York, New York: Rodale Press, Inc./St. Martin's Press, 1997).

Eagle, C. and Harish, J. "Elements of Ppain and Music: The Aio Connection," *Journal of the American Association for Music Therapists*, Vol. 7, Issue 1 (1988): 15-27.

Gardner, W. and Licklider, J. "Auditory Analgesia in Dental Operations," *Journal of the American Dental Association*, 59 (1959): 1144–50.

Gardner, W.; Licklider, J.; and Weisz, A. "Suppression of Pain by Sound," *Science*, 132 (1960): 32–33.

Godley, C. "The Use of Music in Pain Clinics," *Music Therapy Perspectives*, 4 (1987): 24–28.

Grout, D. J. *A History of Western Music, Rev.* (New York, New York: W. W. Norton & Company, Inc., 1973).

Hay, L. *Heal Your Body: The Mental Causes for Physical Illness and the Metaphysical Way to Overcome Them.* (Carlsbad, Calif.: Hay House, 1984).

Hilliard, R. "The Effects of Music Therapy on the Quality and Length of Life of People Diagnosed with Terminal Cancer," *Journal of Music Therapy*, Vol. 40, Issue 2 (2003): 113–37.

Horden, P. (Ed.) *Music as Medicine: The History of Music Therapy since Antiquity.* (Burlington, Vermont: Ashgate Publishing Company, 2000).

Kenny, D. and Faunce, G. "The Impact of Group Singing on Mood, Coping, and Perceived Pain in Chronic Pain Patients Attending a Multidisciplinary Pain Clinic," *Journal of Music Therapy*, Vol. 41, Issue 3 (2004): 241–58.

Standley, J. "Clinical Applications of Music and Chemotherapy: The Effects of Nausea and Emesis," *Music Therapy Perspectives*, Vol. 10, Issue 1 (1992), 27–35.

Taylor, D. *Biomedical Foundations of Music as Therapy*. (St. Louis, Mo.: MMB Music, Inc., 1997)

Valone, T. *Bioelectromagnetic Healing: A Rationale for Its Use*. (Washington, D.C.: Integrity Research Institute, 2000).

Walworth, D. "The Effect of Preferred Music Genre Selection versus Preferred Song Selection on Experimentally Induced Anxiety Levels," *Journal of Music Therapy*, Volume 40, Issue 1 (2003): 2–14.

Warburg, O. "On the Origin of Cancer Cells," *Science*, 123 (1956): 309.

Wigram, T.; Pedersen, I.; and Bonde, L. *A Comprehensive Guide to Music Therapy: Theory, Clinical Practice, Research and Training*. (London: Jessica Kingsley Publishers, Inc., 2002)

Wigram, T.; Saperston, B.; and West, R. (Eds.) *The Art and Science of Music Therapy: A Handbook*. (Rutledge, 1995).

Wolfe, D. "Pain Rehabilitation and Music Therapy," *Journal of Music Therapy*, Vol. 15, Issue 4 (1978): 162–78.

Zimmerman, L.; Pozehl, B.; Duncan, K.; and Schmitz, R. "Effects of Music in Patients Who Had Chronic Cancer Pain," *Western Journal of Nursing Research*, 11 (1989): 209–309.

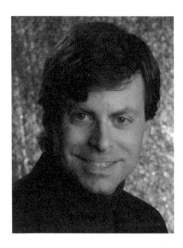 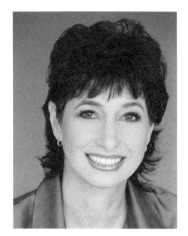

Howard Richman is a pianist, composer, music teacher, and sound researcher. He has been blending his advanced music training and intuitive awareness to create healing music since 1982. He is a pioneer in the entrainment approach to sound-healing techniques. He holds a bachelor of arts degree in piano performance from UCLA and a master of fine arts degree from California Institute of the Arts, where he served on the faculty for three years. Mr. Richman's specialty is to help people break through their most stubborn obstacles with unconventional solutions. He performs and speaks throughout the United States and abroad. He lives in Los Angeles.

Judy Nelson is a board-certified music therapist and speech language pathologist. She is one of the founders of the Music Therapy Wellness Center at California State University, Northridge, where she is an associate professor. She holds a bachelor of arts degree in music performance from California State University, Hayward and a master of science degree in communication disorders from California State University, Northridge. She is also an instructor in meditation, guided imagery, and stress reduction. Her specialty is integrating music therapy, guided imagery, and relaxation to music, meditation, and stress-management techniques for adults with chronic illness and pain. Ms. Nelson is also a professional vocalist who performs and lives in Los Angeles.